Gastro-Esophageal Reflux Disease: A Self-Help Guide

Dietary Treatment of Gastro-Esophageal Reflux

Constantin Panow

Copyright 2012
All rights reserved.

"All ailment starts in the gut".
Hippocrates (460-370BC)

CONTENTS

Disclaimer

The author and publisher decline responsibility about any injury or deleterious effect that could result from misinterpretation or wrong understanding and application of this text.

This short guide shouldn't be understood as a substitute for professional care by a gastroenterologist or another specialist.

Its aim is to fill a gap between professional literature and individual care by physicians.

It is a self- help guide aiming at better care for this disease.

Key words

Gastro- esophageal reflux, lower esophageal sphincter insufficiency (stomach inlet insufficiency), reflux esophagitis, hiatal herniation, gastro- esophageal reflux disease, GERD.

PREVALENCE

Gastro- esophageal reflux is a frequent complaint. About a third of the population of industrialized countries suffers from GERD on and off.

ANATOMY

The anatomical substrate for GERD consists in a faulty ligament restraint of movements of distal esophagus. (I e ligaments linking distal esophagus to diaphragm.)

Its full- blown image is hiatal herniation, which is the term frequently used for convenience's sake in this text.

Hiatal herniation causes incompetency of lower esophageal sphincter (gastric inlet), and thus allows stomach content to reflux in lower esophagus.

1.

How to be sure, you have gastro esophageal reflux

– Identifying acid in your mouth at night.

– Burning sensation or frank pain in upper abdomen and lower chest: in the middle, going up towards the throat, worst at night or after a heavy meal, relieved by upright position.

– If you are not sure about your symptoms, going to a doctor's office is the simplest way to ascertain about them.

– Symptoms are greatly improved by antacid medication.

- Chronic cough at night can be the only manifestation of GERD.

2.

Factors which determine this illness

–Family history: most of the time hiatal herniation is a family flaw.

–Environmental factors and alimentary habits, the single most important of all is overweight and recent weight gain.

- Decompensation of GERD with reflux esophagitis can be triggered by any inflammatory event. Many infectious agents can be involved. Though most of the time it is the result of minor viral infection of the gastro- intestinal tract.

- As such viral infections go otherwise unrecognized, are very frequent, and there is no specific treatment for them, most medical authorities refuse investigations of triggering agent and treat symptomatically.

The main goal of this booklet is to help you avoiding major alimentary hygiene mistakes, which can worsen gastro- esophageal reflux.

3.

Why is it important?

Although antacid medication is efficient to counteract acidity and diminish pain, it doesn't correct anatomy and can't prevent you from choking at night because of a heavy meal. Sometimes this could be even a death- triggering event. Especially if you are under action of alcohol or sleeping medicine, which diminish coughing reflex on food entering the trachea.

Although gastric anti- secretory drugs are safe, full innocuity of long- term antacid medication hasn't been proved. Generally: the less medication you use, the better!

To this consideration comes price, which is still relatively high for potent antacids.

Though efficient antacid medication is available since many years, practitioners still see on- and- off patients who respond poorly to this conventional treatment and develop long- term complications.

COMPLICATIONS

-Are of 3 kinds:

The first is observed on endoscopy and biopsy as mucosal gastric metaplasia of distal esophagus, so called Barrett's disease.

(This means that distal esophagus is constantly bathed by gastric juice and with time changes it's covering for a more appropriate gastric mucosa.)

This complication ends with time in a more serious disease, which is called endo-brachy-esophagus, which means foreshortening of esophagus.

(In this condition the whole wall of the tubing is involved with sclerotic changes.)

After years, Barrett's esophagus is also at risk for developing cancer of lower esophagus, most of the time adenocarcinoma.

Thus, present short dietetic instruction shouldn't be understood as an alternative to medical therapy, but rather as a complement to conventional treatment of GERD.

Operative correction of hiatal herniation is proposed only for complex cases, which can't be solved otherwise, and most authorities don't resort to surgery in the big majority of patients. Besides, surgery is frequently inefficient to correct appropriately anatomy (30% failure in big series).

4.

HABITS

- Which worsen gastro- esophageal reflux: chocolate, alcohol, tobacco, hot chili, pepper, and yogurt eaten at night.

Some medication is also poorly tolerated in the presence of GERD: anti- inflammatory drugs, aspirin, even at low dose, Vitamin D...

Most important factor being: Eating late a heavy meal, just before going to bed.

5.

STRESS AND ENVIRONMENT.

- Whole body sun exposition during holidays. In such a situation you must have always some strong antacids, to take early at night and cut extra acid production.

MEDICATION

Strong antacid drug is in fact gastric anti-secretory medication, and is of two types:

- H2 receptor antagonist (cimetidine and ranitidine)

- Proton pump inhibitor (esomeprazole, lansoprazole, omeprazole, pantoprazole and rabeprazole)

6.

RULES TO EATING HYGIENE.

A.The bigger the evening- meal, the worst gastro- esophageal reflux at night.

B. More you eat during the whole day; worst are problems of reflux.

In fact, this depends rather on discrepancy between energy expenditure and food intake.

I e you can eat lots more without trouble if you practice strenuous sports or work and burn efficiently the calories you ingest.

7. Explanation: There is little risk of having gastro- esophageal reflux with an empty stomach.

Eating supper early enough in the evening would provide your stomach enough time to empty before bedtime.

The stomach empties at a specific pace, which is regulated by inner neuro- humoral mechanisms.

AVERAGE ½ EMPTYING FOR SOLIDS IS ¾ H.

AVERAGE ½ EMPTYING FOR LIQUIDS IS ¼ H.

(Prof. Edouard Loizeau, Geneva University Hospital)

These averages are though subject to enormous variations depending on several factors.

Aim of this guide is to make you understand those factors and alleviate symptoms of incomplete stomach emptying at night.

Fastening, though it is warranty for an empty stomach, is not a solution, as binge eating, and unevenness of meals promotes the worst exacerbation of gastric acidity secretion and is the main cause for true dyspepsia.

Advice: if your stomach is empty at night, but you feel a burning sensation because of excess acidity secretion, before taking any medicine, you can try following tip: drink just a glass of water. This would dilute stomach acidity and permit stomach content to empty into small bowel. Wait for it a few minutes in upright position.

This presentation happens most of the time because you have overestimated your nutritional needs during the day and have eaten more than necessary (more calories ingested than you have burnt during the day).

Every person needs a certain amount of energy every day, which should be taken as food, to allow for normal functioning of the body.

The way you would distribute these daily meals

and the kind of food you take before going to bed would determine evolution of your gastro-esophageal reflux.

- Heavy meals during the whole day, whose energetic content exceeds present needs of your organism would slow down stomach emptying at night.

Once you have understood by personal experience the goal of this guide, you would be able to eat only one meal during the whole day and even take it just before going to bed.

Still, eating only one meal per day is an unhealthy habit, to be avoided as far as possible.

But your aim should be optimal mastering of this diet, which would give you more freedom in your professional life.

As a matter of fact, every one of us has experienced on- and - off a busy day with no time for a break.

But at first, you must start little by little to make yourself familiar with the principles of this guide.

At the beginning it would be more expedient to eat your main meal at lunchtime and breakfast, to have to add only a small amount of energy supply at night.

This strategy makes mistakes more easily avoidable.

Another point is that reflux esophagitis has tendency to manifest itself in middle age.

-Mainly because of weight gain.

-Consider that after 50, your body needs much less calories, unless, of course, you are a heavy-duty worker. Many authorities consider that after 50 two meals a day are enough. (All metabolic functions of your organism become slower with aging.)

-Some sports activity would keep you in shape and could make more easy dealing with GERD.

Understanding what quantity of food your body needs for your daily work is probably the most important point in the whole learning process.

MACRO-NUTRIMENTS

There are three main components to any meal (called macro-nutrients).

1. – proteins: composed of amino- acids

2. – lipids: composed of fatty acids, saturated or poly-, unsaturated.

3. – Carbohydrates: composed of Fiber-carbohydrates and Starches, complex or simple sugars.

Different dishes have a different composition of these three main components.

EXAMPLES

Meat: high protein content, but also frequently a lot of lipids (fatty acids), varying after quality of product.

Fish: High protein content; high quality lipids, frequently low amount, much lower lipid content than that of meat.

Cheese: proteins and lipids.

Butter, oil: lipids.

Bread: mainly Starches.
Pasta products: mainly Starches.
Rice: mainly Starches.
Potatoes: mainly Starches.
Carrots: mainly Fiber-Carbohydrates.
Red beet: high Starches content.
Cereals other than wheat: also, mainly Starches.

In contradistinction to old views, white bread, pasta, rice, potatoes, and other cereals are mainly to be considered not as slow sugars, but as fast sugars.

Only a few minutes after their ingestion, they are available as glucose in your blood.

But if you add some lipids to them, you slow down stomach emptying, and convert them to "slow sugars".

In this regard you can consider glucose index of macro-nutrients (but this is of secondary importance in this diet, though low glucose index, below 6, can certainly be better handled by the stomach, and slow down less stomach emptying than a meal with high glucose index.)

COMBINATION OF MACRO-NUTRIMENTS

Composition of your meal would determine largely pace of stomach emptying.

Ingested meal interacts with receptors in proximal small bowel, which trigger release of intestinal hormones.

These ones determine tonus and contraction of gastric outlet (pylorus) and gastric wall muscles.

Hence composition of ingested meal determines pace of stomach emptying.

If you mix all three components in equal amounts, proteins, lipids and sugars, stomach emptying would be slowest.

Your aim is not to slow down stomach emptying at supper by eating a « bomb » of energy, but to avoid disagreeable feeling of an empty stomach at night, by providing some energy that is due to your body after a strenuous working day.

If you take only one kind of the 3 main components, stomach emptying would be fastest, and you would avoid reflux.

SLOWEST EMPTYING OCCURS WITH LIPIDS > SUGARS > PROTEINS.

As you see from the table above, most products that you buy in supermarket are not pure and contain already at least two of the three basic components.

This way, because most food that you can buy contains already two of three main components, all you can do is choosing between limited numbers of possibilities.

You should know that you would have the second biggest problem mixing sugars with lipids, this composition having the most relaxing effect on lower esophageal sphincter (stomach inlet).

The other factor that determines intensity of gastro esophageal reflux being tonus of lower esophageal sphincter.

You would have the least problems by mixing proteins with lipids. For instance, some fish at night with salad would be the ideal evening meal for you and your family.

Being limited by products that you buy, you should still do your best at avoiding too much of either component.

For instance, if you choose to eat meat at supper, don't forget that adding oil to it is just necessary for cooking and to make your meal palatable.

Lipids are the highest energy components of the three. Every g of lipids is worth 9 kcal, while every g of sugars is worth only 4 kcal. As proteins on an energetic basis can by transformed in glucose, their caloric value is also 4.

You shouldn't exaggerate by adding too much oil, as lipids are between the most potent relaxants of lower esophageal sphincter, and they slow down also most efficiently emptying of your stomach.

This means also, you should give up a dessert at night, as this would be the main dish to promote problems with your hiatal herniation.
Choosing copious sweet dessert after a normal meal is the best insurance to spend a sleepless night.

Carbohydrates as a single meal are second best choice, but it would always be second best, because stomach emptying after such a meal is slow and relaxation of lower esophageal sphincter intense.
If you choose Carbs, you can, and must limit to a greater extent lipid content.
This is also very important in regard of the fact that this would be always a second-best choice for a healthy supper.
If so, if for instance you choose to eat only some

bread at supper, don't mix it with any proteins, as this would substantially worsen problems.

For instance, vegetable soup with some bread represents a very good solution for supper.

Another solution is to choose black bread (whole grain), rather than white, which contains slow sugars (with lower glucose index).

This way you can add more safely some oil or butter to make your meal tastier.

Do not forget to eat bread or potatoes at breakfast and lunch, as this would provide you with fast available calories, but avoid this kind of component in the evening.

If you have been working especially hard, do not wait till evening comes to boost some energy to your body, as it needs it.

But do it early before supper, for instance at 4- 5 pm, and if possible, by eating fast sugars, for instance bread or potatoes or rice alone.

Remember, the main calorie- support your brain uses is pure sugar- glucose.

Recent evidence points to the fact that this organ can adapt, as well as the whole body, to Ketone Bodies.

(Glucose body reserves are very limited in quantity. They consist of glycogen, mostly in the liver, with a smaller reserve in your muscles.)

If you move slower, at a steady pace, work is

done as well by muscles and brain using some lipid-energy rich support.

If you feel jittery or any other sign of hypoglycemia, remember to provide your body with Carbs first, and the sooner the better.

HYPOGLYCEMIA

Hypoglycemia manifests with rapid pulse, sweating, paleness, and tremor.

Hypoglycemia is usually expected if energy expenditures have been higher than energy provided by meals. Though, sometimes you would become hypoglycemic unexpectedly, without obvious reason. One explanation for such an event is viral illness. Bacterial infection is most of the time obvious, accompanied by high fever and other complaints. Viral illness, on the contrary, goes frequently unrecognized, though higher energy expenditures, and resulting hypoglycemia can be the only manifestation.

SPORTS & FITNESS

Exercise as such promotes faster emptying of stomach, because of higher energy expenditure.

Though, remember that strenuous exercise can block stomach emptying for a while.

Exercising in recumbent position with a full stomach can heavily worsen GERD.

Sports of any kind can solve your GERD problems on their own.

Examination of sumo fighters in Japan showed that a diet in excess combined with strenuous exercise deposits fat mainly subcutaneously and not as visceral fat (intra-abdominal).

As intra-abdominal fat is the main promoter of GERD in most cases, any kind of sports, be it aerobics or Anaerobic on a continuous basis can solve or improve your GERD problem.

Remember, though, if you start with such a program, that exercise in a recumbent state can exert a reverse effect on GERD.

Exercise always, if in a recumbent state, with little stomach filling. (The best is while fasting). But this can be appreciated only on individual basis. Personal experience with it is most important than all, and this guide directs you only to general rules applicable to this topic.

Sports augments also glycogen muscle storage if practiced regularly and avoids to a big extent hypoglycemia in aging population.

Your aim should be to have an empty stomach when you go to sleep, or almost, with the least relaxation of lower esophageal sphincter and the least acid content in the stomach.

MISTAKES

If you do a mistake; this would happen frequently at beginning and seldom after several years of practicing with this diet.

There is still one last thing you can try before taking some medicine.

Lie- down on your left side and stay in this position for the first part of the night, till your stomach empties.

In left lateral position stomach content exercises traction on gastro- esophageal junction and makes lower esophageal sphincter more efficient.

Left lateral position tends to straighten any hiatal herniation, if present.

The fuller the stomach, the stronger traction is exercised by its content.

But this would be efficient only as long as you haven't relaxed lower esophageal sphincter exceedingly with some energetic food, and as long your stomach is not too full to bulge content into its upper part.

GREEN SALAD

Green salad by itself doesn't exercise any substantial adverse effect on half- emptying of stomach, or relaxation of lower esophageal sphincter.

Though, as gastric secretion contains the strongest known acid, chlorohydric acid, HCL:

Any additive food has a tampon- effect on acidity; and if relatively neutral chemically, exerts an action of simple dilution of stomach juice.

As such, salad, as well as any neutral ballast matter, should be favored for an evening meal (aimed at reducing acid secretion).

The 3 main components, proteins, sugars and lipids, stimulate all three stomach acid secretion.

If you eat a meal without useful ballast matter, you take a bigger risk of ending with excessive acid content during the night.

On the other hand, constipation has also an adverse effect on gastro-esophageal reflux.

Taking some bulk during evening meals in the form of salad also counteracts constipation, and by this way can also have a positive effect on your symptoms.

Some people suffer from GERD mainly because they are constipated and thick bowel content reaches such proportions that hiatal herniation manifests, for similar space reasons as in weight gain.

This of course if you consider all composition of a salad, which can contain for instance red beet, or corn, near to pure sugar.
- Or oil as a dressing.
- Or eggs or other proteins, already mixed with fat.

As matter of fact one of the best solutions of a supper or evening meal can be offered in the presentation of a salad.

It can contain shrimps, fish, eggs, cheese, or anything else you enjoy.

ROLE OF LIQUIDS

Liquids, neither don't influence heavily by themselves pace of stomach emptying.

The only fact you must consider if you are very thirsty just before bedtime:

- is that a very full stomach, because of excessive content, can make lower esophageal sphincter inefficient, based on simple mechanistic rules.

Liquids by themselves don't exercise a tampon effect on acidity. They just dilute it, but don't interact with it as ballast matter does.

Once you have gained experience with this regime, you would discover you could eat whatever you like at supper.

In fact, it is all a matter of experience.

The devil is in the detail.

The substance of this diet is in the amount of each compound and in the sequence of its ingestion.

When you have become familiar with physiology of your stomach, you would be even able to eat only one meal during the whole day, and this at night, just before going to bed.

But for doing so, you must have gathered quite a lot of experience.

At the beginning it is wiser to eat a small meal at supper, and eat it early enough, so the stomach can have time to empty till bedtime.

31

STRATIFICATION OF FOOD

Though people think that all different dishes that they eat at one meal are mixed in the stomach, reality is far from that.

As a matter of fact, only liquids mix between themselves in the stomach.

All solids remain stratified in the order in which you ingest them.

Few nutriments are digested already in the stomach, and even fewer are absorbed in this organ.

(Apart from alcohol and water, which can be absorbed to a non- negligible percentage in the stomach, everything else is absorbed in the small bowel.)

This means that if you respect a strict order in which you eat different plates, you can take a whole supper containing all three main components in one meal.

But until you have mastered easier stages of this diet, this principle would remain for you only theory.

If everything else fails, be sure you have still some potent antacid medicines, as a last resort.

In cases of reflux esophagitis, which most of the time is promoted by viral gastro- intestinal inflammation, you would need your medicine anyway.

And you would need it as long, until esophagitis heals.

Then only you can return to your diet, as it is rather a preventive measure, than a healing procedure.

With time you would discover, that instead of the packages of medicine you were eating, you would need a potent antacid only on a few occasions during the whole year.

SELF-EVALUATION

How would you know whether your regime is efficient at controlling GERD?

This is quite easy to accomplish. To be sure about results and avoid complications, you can lead a record about GERD bouts.

How many per month?

How long in duration?

How free are you from inflammation between bouts of disease?

Of course this can be accomplished by a professional, but no medical worker can provide a better job than yourself in this evaluation.

To my opinion this task should be considered a complement to any medical care by a doctor.

Drinking strong alcohol or eating spicy food or sour food lets you feel quite reliably whether there is some inflammation of lower esophagus. Strength of pain on GERD bouts informs you also reliably about degree of inflammation.

(Exception to this rule might be if you suffer from diabetes mellitus since a long time or have other neuropathy, which doesn't allow you to feel pain. Diabetes also promotes gastroparesis, in which situation emptying of the stomach might be exceptionally prolonged.)

As stated previously GERD manifests frequently after weight gain.

This implies you should also take care of your weight problem, before being able to solve the one of your hiatal herniation.

CAUTION

-If you suffer from GERD, scuba diving is decisively to be avoided.

Hiatal herniation also prevents athletes from performing correctly in most swimming disciplines, as the small column of water above swimmer's head, when he expires air, exercises sufficient pressure to send air down the esophagus and in the stomach, through its incompetent inlet.

Little considered by professionals and afflicted individuals as well, this is probably main cause of death while Scuba Diving.

Not having oriented a second thought to this particularity, if you are under water, you do not know how to react!

Trying to swallow liquid back into the stomach is probably the most fatal mistake. (Risk of Broncho-Aspiration) Spitting everything that comes up can be lifesaving.

As simple as that!

If you have the habit of an afternoon nap, you should apply this regime also to your meal at lunchtime, or you should give up sleeping in the afternoon.

EVENING MEALS PROPOSALS

Different meal- proposals for supper:

1.

Proteins and lipids

-Fish and salad: No rice, bread, Italian pasta, corn, potatoes, or other cereals. Instead, you can season your fish and salad as you wish with butter or oil.

But prefer rather vegetable oil, as it is healthier, and don't forget to also switch oil origin from time to time, which makes cooking more palatable, and adds new flavors to it. Don't forget your brain, which is nourished best with different kinds of vegetable oils, containing all different essential polyunsaturated fatty acids (sunflower, peanut, pumpkin seeds, grape- seeds, thistle, and walnut, to name only a few sources of vegetable oils).

-Shrimp cocktail, (but applies to crab and lobster meat as well.)

As shrimps contain mostly proteins which are very slowly absorbed, you can add any kind of salad you wish to it. The stomach considers this kind of proteins almost as "salad", and doesn't delay considerably it's emptying because of their presence, which allows more freedom in preparing this kind of supper.

-White chicken meat. Add salad as you like but avoid strictly Starches- containing components like corn and other cereals.

-Meat of any kind and salad.

Possible combination, but you should pay attention to quantity of meat. Better meat quality, i.e. low-fat one allows to increase quantity, but this only to a certain extent which is very individual. Appreciation needs a lot of experience, so this plate is not considered a beginner's plate with this diet. Of course, by no means add any rice, bread or equivalent combined Starches!

A sugary dessert with this kind of meal is the deadliest combination ever for a person with hiatal herniation.

-Cheese and salad.

Also, a possible combination, but needs same care with choice of quality and quantity, as for meat. Prefer fresh cheese, type cottage cheese in place of cooked yellow cheese, but this is only a relative incentive! Most important is probably quantity.

Prohibit any kind of fast sugars, contained especially in desserts, as these relax indefinitely lower esophageal sphincter (stomach inlet)! Limit sugar in sweet beverages as well, to one or two dice! Consider soft drinks contain a huge amount of simple sugars, very unhealthy drinks!

Salad as combination is intended as green salad, but may be replaced or added with cauliflower of any kind, broccoli, cabbage, green, string or snap beans (not old beans)

FOOD INTOLERANCE

An aspect to pay attention to, is alimentary intolerance or « allergy », a phenomenon better understood since about 40 years.

We are still at the beginning of this knowledge. We have learnt for instance by recent experience that some vegetables can be extremely allergenic, a category which can render difficult intestinal treatment and absorption of meal.

For instance, celery and hazelnuts are two components to which many people are allergic. But many other alimentary components can be allergenic in your precise case, so you must always ask yourself how well you digest each vegetable separately, if you intend to include it in an evening meal.

According to present state of medicine, about 30 % of people are allergic to nutritional compounds. As knowledge increases, this percentage can only grow.

If you are not sure about a compound, just omit it from your supper recipe, as such a meal can need much too long to be dealt with in your body.

Stomach emptying can be delayed extremely because of meal intolerance or allergy.

Suspicious vegetables in this regard are soft peppers, onions, cabbage, cauliflower, and to some extent tomatoes. This last vegetable can be better tolerated if it is cooked or pealed, but you should always consider quantity.

If you are not certain about tolerance, limit quantity!

Some fruit is also heavy at supper for similar reasons, one example being strawberries, regardless of allergy.

Old beans

Independent of color and type (green, brown, white, yellow, big, small), they all contain slow Carbs and proteins. If you add any kind of lipids to make this plate palatable, you have an explosive combination. This is a high energy meal to reserve, if possible, for lunch, and avoid or eat only in limited amount of it at night.

If you still choose it as an evening meal, avoid any kind of bread or similar food with it, a combination which can extend digestion indefinitely. Do not add meat or other high protein food to it.

Lentils

Same considerations as for old beans. These two are very similar components, but of high-quality everyday meals. To reserve, if possible, for lunch, or breakfast for heavy body workers.

Green peas

This is a very neutral ingredient, but needs cooking, because of its Lectins content. Can be added to green salad or substituted for it as an evening meal. Fiber-Carbohydrates and little protein content usually well tolerated.

Mushrooms

Can replace green salad, mainly ballast, containing complex Sugars, which need special bacteria in the intestines to be absorbed.

Consider uncommon species can be less well tolerated, on individual basis. Some people lack specific enzymes to digest them, which manifests invariably as diarrhea after their ingestion.

2.

Combination of complex
Sugars and lipids

This combination is second best after proteins and lipids, as it promotes a stronger relaxation of lower esophageal sphincter.

If you choose it, avoid adding any proteins of any kind or nature, as this would lead you to the worst choice of combining all three main components (proteins + lipids + sugars)

This combination represents many possibilities in which the main limitation is quantity.

Examples

-Stuffed vine leaves with rice.

-Stuffed cabbage leaves with rice.

-Bread and butter (Avoid any cheese at supper, as it contains proteins!)

-Potatoes and butter or preferably oil (consider added nutritive value of polyunsaturated lipids which should be preferred to saturated lipids!)

-Corn salad. Any green salad or equivalent would do. Remember not to add any proteins, especially tuna or other fish, as by doing so you would end with the worst combination (proteins, lipids in the salad sauce and starches)!

Salad can be added with usual limitations concerning certain products as above.

- Italian pasta: cannelloni, spaghetti, macaroni, or similar food. Avoid meat or cheese ingredients, which frequently belong to a true Italian dish!

3.

Different

Substitutes of green salad

-Soya: a very neutral ingredient of traditional Asian cuisine, usually well tolerated, containing slow sugars and proteins, which can be added to any meal with little limitation, in the same way as green salad.

-Radishes: strong taste limits usually quantity by itself.

This ingredient (radishes) exercises a positive effect on gastric acidity, inhibiting acid secretion by the stomach. Can be added to an evening meal without limitation for this purpose.

-Spinach: can replace green salad advantageously without negative incentive. Endives: can also replace green salad without negative advice.

-Courgetti: a very useful vegetable, containing slow carbs, preferably cooked than raw. No negative limitation. Very well tolerated usually.

-Asparagus: in the same way can replace green salad or spinach and bring variety to your cooking. Very well tolerated. No real limitation.

-Egg plants: contains slow sugars. Served cooked, especially fried.

Constitutes traditional eastern European cuisine with a sauce of yoghurt. This last is the sole limitation for this traditional dish, as yoghurt also contains proteins to a non-negligible level, and acts by itself as a potent relaxation agent of lower esophageal sphincter. Yoghurt in the traditional dish can be replaced at night by another sauce. Soya-sauce or even mayonnaise, avoiding any adding of proteins, the dish being by itself already cooked usually in oil and being heavy because of this. You can add bread or rice or potatoes but pay attention again to quantity of these last ingredients!

-Artichoke: stimulates bile secretion. Rather dietetic dish, which can replace advantageously green salad.

-Avocado: high lipid content. Can replace green salad spin some dishes, but always consider its high energy, 1 g of lipids being equivalent to 9 kcal, while

1 g of sugars is equivalent to 4 kcal.

-Bamboo sprouts: can replace green salad in all regards.

-Brussels sprouts: like cabbage, sometimes a source of food intolerance, to discuss on individual level. Otherwise contains slow complex sugars, very slowly absorbed in intestines. Decisive advantage towards cabbage is probably shorter cooking necessary to make it palatable.

-Celery salad: very high-quality dish for those who are not allergic to it.

-Cucumber: little nutritive value. Brings mainly microelements to the body. Can replace green salad in all regards.

-Fennel: stimulates bile juice secretion. Very dietetic dish. Can be added advantageously to any meal.

-Leek: similar disadvantage as onions, to a lesser degree. Frequent cause of food intolerance.

-Lettuce: almost same as green salad.

-Okra: seldom food intolerance. High nutritive value. Few disadvantages. Can be added almost to any dish at supper.

-Peppers: to be avoided at supper. Heavy meal, probably because of high level of intolerance in general population.

-Spinach: almost like green salad. Different trace elements.

-Squash: difficult to prepare. Rather low- quality substitute for green salad.

4.

Dessert

-As a dessert any fruit can do. The only aspect that needs consideration is sugar content of the fruit you intend to have as dessert.

-Apples, though presenting little problems of intolerance, because of their high percentage of combined and simple sugars, digested to some extent in gastric juice to glucose and fructose, relax lower esophageal sphincter most intensely, and thus should be limited in quantity and pealed.

(Consider gastric juice contains also swallowed saliva, one component of it being ptyalin, an enzyme that splits complex sugars.)

-Similar consideration can be applied to grapes. Any added sugar is heavily paid for with extreme relaxation of lower esophageal sphincter.

-Pears are better tolerated, but because of laxative effect should be limited in number.

-For every other fruit the only variable that counts is sweetness, which is in direct proportion to simple sugar content. As there are many different varieties of fruit, it is essential that you train yourself to appreciate simple sugars content after sweetness of ingredient.

-On the contrary to people's beliefs, citrus fruit, like oranges, pomelos, mandarins, clementines and grapefruit, though considered to be most digestible at breakfast or lunch and "heavy" at supper, have little adverse effect on lower esophageal sphincter relaxation and stomach emptying.

-Sour fruit is a problem only if reflux esophagitis is already at hand. In this situation you need your doctor, and of course potent antacids, till inflammation subsides.

You feel burning sensation on passage of sour fruit through gastric inlet when there is inflammation. – Can be used as diagnostic tool to appreciate effectiveness of hygienic measures and anti-secretory medicine.

-Bananas should be avoided at supper, unless they constitute your main dish. If you add them as a dessert, unless the first plate consists also of complex sugars, they would add carbs to a meal of proteins in a very unpleasant sense, delaying indefinitely stomach emptying.

FEASTS

Eating only one meal a day after dusk, represents a real challenge for people with hiatal herniation.

If I have some advice to give in this context: I propose to ask for help a professional, as a somatic illness like hiatal herniation, needs a special consideration by religious authority and can be exonerated from strict alimentary and religious rules.

If you still want to proceed with such a constriction to general alimentary rules, to my opinion a rather unhealthy diet for people with hiatal herniation, this is still feasible, but needs a special training and experience, which can be gained only by thorough observance of easier above guidelines.

As a first proposition, I would suggest treating first main somatic need by drinking daily amount of beverages, soup, cold and warm drinks, which can contain simple sugars to replenish first body needs.

Then, eating complex Carbs in the form of rice, bread, mill, pasta, potatoes, which would provide your organism with first needed energy lost during daily work.

The main advice would be to take enough time to restore your body.

Consider you have jumped two or three normal meals during the day!

Take at least three- four times normal meal's time to restore your body. Do not be in a hurry! Indeed, if it's a feast, that's how you can enjoy it most.

Reserve quality products like proteins for the end but think about avoiding mixing of foods in the stomach by choosing liquids at the beginning and solids at the end.

Again, use general rules of above guidelines by avoiding mixing proteins, fast sugars, and lipids in the same meal.

If you start with a mixture of complex carbs as bread or cereals, avoid mixing them with oily stuff or meat.

Eat enough salad in between to prevent mixture of two different meals, and keep proteins, which would restore your muscle and all tissues, for the end, possibly with a bit of oily ingredients, which would provide you with long term energy for the next day!

And before all, consider quantity, taking enough time to ingest all this complex regime!

If you must keep such a rhythm for several weeks, this is the worst time to deal with reflux esophagitis, so don't experiment new rules or dishes you haven't tried before.

During normal part of the year, you should

gather recipes that you have tried under normal conditions, and resort to them during religious feast, but avoid completely new experimentation with which you have no knowledge.

This kind of regime is possible for a person suffering from hiatal herniation, but it is not easy or simple.

A thorough knowledge of stomach physiology is required to be successful.

PLEASURE

Finally: Consider that a meal, and especially an evening meal must be a pleasurable experience.

To some extent Epicurean Philosophy plays a central role in stomach emptying.

If your company needs some alcohol to enjoy thoroughly this occasion, don't hesitate to introduce a small "mistake" into your daily routine.

But remember, rather choose quality than quantity, and your hiatal herniation won't bother you at night, especially if you have enjoyed your evening!

STOMACH CANCER

This one had encumbered Japanese and European population for centuries because mainly of the habit consisting of eating raw vegetables with little fat mixed.

Change in nutritional regime with high protein ingestion has heavily improved odds.

Remains prevalence of adenocarcinoma at distal esophagus, related to GERD. Obesity Epidemic worsens this parameter.

EXPOSURE TO COLD

With recent interest in Cold Baths has become evident the fact of reduction in visceral fat with such a practice.

Thermic shock takes a toll every year in imprudent practitioners.

A softer method is increasing vegetal oil and fish consume at the expense of other animal fat.

This also tends to redistribute favorably body fat.

WEBSITE

If you have any questions or look for advice with this topic, please feel free to write in my blog: www.thenopillshealthprospect.com

Made in the USA
Monee, IL
07 July 2026

56552678R00036